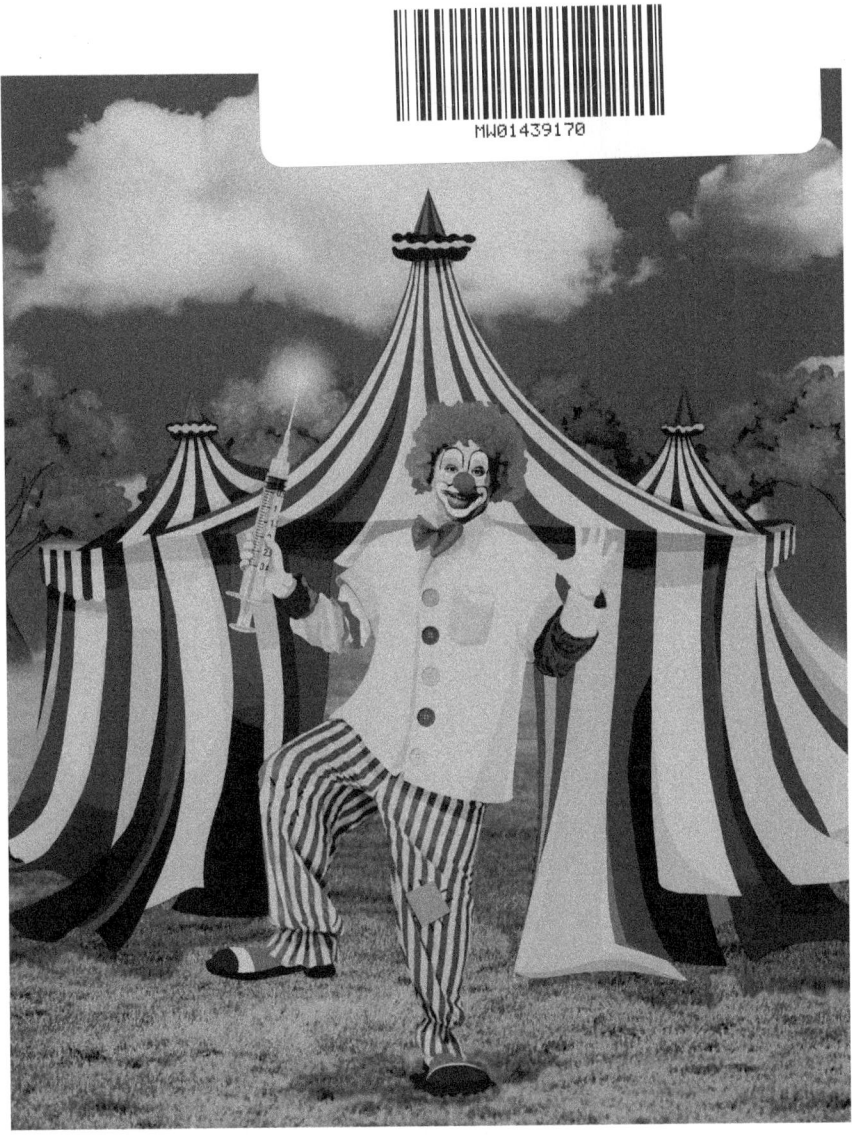

"Circus Tent" Illustrated by Thomas Cetnarowski

dfd
BELOW THE CIRCUS TENT

BELOW THE CIRCUS TENT

Dealing with Tough Times

JESSICA WEGRZYNOWSKI

Below The Circus Tent
Jessica Wegrzynowski

COPYRIGHT ©2023 Jessica Wegrzynowski
All Rights Reserved
Improper use of this publication, reproduction, distribution etc. is restricted.

ISBN: 978-1-7380601-0-8

DEDICATION

Dedicated to all the hospitals I've stayed in and its wonderful medical staff. Thank you for taking good care of me and for never giving up on me.

ACKNOWLEDGEMENTS

I would like to thank:

My parents, Margret and Adam Wegrzynowski, for their love, support, guidance, patience and for always being by my side during good times and bad.

My sister, Malvina Wegrzynowski, for her love, encouragement, advice, and her eternal faith in me.

Thomas Cetnarowski for his Circus Tent illustration.

Misty Ciarniello for editing and for her encouragement.

The entire Tri-Cities Brain Injury Support Group for their support and for inspiring me.

My friends for their assistance, encouragement, support and advice.

Doctors and nurses for their hard work, devotion, patience and courage.

God for creating me and for the many gifts He has blessed me with.

CONTENTS

Photo Insert — i
Dedication — vii
Acknowledgements — ix

I	Introduction	1
II	A Malicious Melody	2
III	An Amazing Show	4
IV	A Tent Full of Mystery	6
V	Clowning Around	8
VI	Lights, Camera, and Action	10
VII	Taming the Lion	12
VIII	Risky Juggling	14
IX	Balloons	16
X	Walking on A Tightrope	18
XI	Wearing Clown Shoes	20
XII	Circus Express	22
XIII	A Little Bit of Magic	24
XIV	The Giant Elephant in The Room	26
XV	A Timeless Trapeze Act	28

XVI	Sword Swallowing	30
XVII	Human Cannonball	32
XVIII	Final Words	34

About The Author   35

CHAPTER I

Introduction

While growing up, I had a very normal childhood. I was energetic, physically active, bold, and outgoing. Also, I loved being the center of attention. There was nothing strange about me, or so I thought until I was fourteen. June 17th, 2003, was a day I will never forget because that's the day my life flipped upside down as I first found out I had a brain injury. Discovering I had a life-threatening injury in my early teens was something no one could have predicted; it was as if it popped up out of thin air. In fact, no one knows how or why I got a brain injury. During this chaotic and confusing time, I would often think my life was becoming a circus. Consequently, during recovery, I wrote several poems about this circus.

CHAPTER II

A Malicious Melody

About The Poem

A Malicious Melody is about the reoccurring headaches I experienced throughout the Spring of 2003. At first, I thought these were normal headaches and so I wasn't too concerned. Eventually, as they occurred more frequently and were almost unbearable, I knew something was not right. At times, these headaches were so intense, I could hardly move a muscle. Hence, I went to several Walk-In Medical Clinics and the doctors who worked there told me these headaches were nothing to worry about.

Poem

A Malicious Melody

No matter where I am, no matter what I do
I hear this unfamiliar music
It dwells deep in my mind
I find it so strange.

During the day, during the night,
I hear this questionable music
When the volume erupts
the fun has begun.

When at school, when at home,
I hear this sketchy music
I try to ignore it but,
it never goes away.

Within my head, within my thoughts
I hear this wonky music
taking over my body,
making me sick.

In the end, in the dark,
I hear this quirky music.
Making it clear
the circus is near.

CHAPTER III

An Amazing Show

About The Poem

As my headaches worsened, eventually so did my body; I had difficulties eating, talking, walking, and breathing. Both my mom and dad got very upset by this so, I told them not to worry. The pain is not so bad; on a scale of one to ten, it's about a five. My parents, however, were not convinced. That's when they took me to the nearest hospital. *An Amazing Show* is about how I tried to put on the "I'm just fine" act for my parents when I knew in my heart and soul I wasn't.

Poem

An Amazing Show

Step right up,
come one,
come all.
Come to the circus
see my amazing act
I must call.
I've sewed all my costumes,
the props are hand-made
Lights are brightly shining
Your ticket's already been paid.
The speakers are booming,
Confetti everywhere.
With hundreds of balloons,
there's no need to share.
My lines have been rehearsed.
No need to be coy.
I begin with a smile and
end with much joy.
A true masterpiece,
everyone does agree.
A show so original.
See a matinee of misery.
I can mask all my feelings.
Make tears be gone
So come see my show,
see this act I can put on.

CHAPTER IV

A Tent Full of Mystery

About The Poem

A Tent Full of Mystery is about the first time I entered a hospital for children. After an MRI scan showed I had a brain tumor I immediately got into an ambulance, which took me to a medical facility more suitable for me. As paramedics wheeled me past the glass automatic doors, I was surprised to see the appearance of this place was dissimilar to any of the hospitals I've seen before. The walls were a warm purple color, the area near the main entrance smelled like sweets and on almost every wall there were pictures of butterflies and teddy bears.

Poem

A Tent Full of Mystery

I stand before a circus tent
with wide, sturdy walls.
Not too sure what to expect,
terror, darkness or worse?
Within seconds my doubts diminish
as I smoothly slip inside.
Marvelous music plays throughout the room
Glitter glistens from way up high.
Everyone here greets me with a smile
making me feel safe and at ease.
A golden balloon is tied to my wrist,
the audience will clap and cheer.
From behind a curtain lions roar
causing my heart to skip a beat.
Bright red lights flash before my eyes.
I am stunned by what I see.
Though these walls seem to sparkle
deep inside I know the truth
This is all one big stage.
A place shouting out to me.

CHAPTER V

Clowning Around

About The Poem

Clowning Around is about the nurses who took care of me. If someone asked me to choose something I like about a hospital, the first thing that would come to mind is the nurses who work there. I cannot imagine what a hospital would be like without nurses. Not only do they help doctors and patients, but they do so with a positive attitude. They are truly strong and courageous. The reason I wrote about clowns is because nurses are often cheerful and try their best to make others smile.

Poem

Clowning Around

Everywhere I look
I see a clown
dancing in circles,
jumping up and down.
They wear silly clothes
nothing too severe.
An enormous smile
painted from ear to ear.
No need for sad faces
just laughter and fun.
Never a dull moment,
sit still and don't run.
When I squeeze on a nose
it is sure to squeak
just like a mouse does
when it tries to speak.
They tell funny jokes,
making me smile
while injecting needles
every once in a while.

CHAPTER VI

Lights, Camera, and Action

About The Poem

Lights, Camera, and Action is about being monitored around the clock. During my hospital stay, nurses (and sometimes doctors) would regularly show up in my room, ask me dozens of questions, take my temperature, and check my heart rate. Nurses would check up on me every half hour during the day and night. Though being monitored twenty-four seven was very helpful and much appreciated, it did quickly become frustrating.

Poem

Lights, Camera, and Action

Curtains rise.
People cheer.
Jaws about to drop.
All eyes on me.
I'm the main attraction.
The center of attention,
so dazzling,
as you can see.
Everyone keeps staring,
cameras always flashing.
So much joy.
It's so sweet.
People seem to adore me,
I know that they all want me,
Life is bliss.
I'm loving it.
Covered up with blankets,
I'm a big sensation
So much envy,
such a thrill.
Fans all around me,
loving every minute,
Come take a peek,
I'm the circus freak.

CHAPTER VII

Taming the Lion

About The Poem

Taming the Lion is about radiation. Due to my brain tumor, doctors advised that I have radiology treatment. During each session, I was required to wear a tight, plastic mask with numerous holes in it while strapped to a bed as a laser pointed at my head for a few minutes. Eventually (after thirty days of treatment) I had another scan, and it showed the radiation had no effect on my injury, which was odd, especially since I was feeling much better. That is when doctors began questioning whether I had been misdiagnosed.

Poem

Taming the Lion

A creature so ferocious
practically begs to be tamed.

Claws capable of commotion.
Teeth sharper than a knife.

I approach with caution
dreading its attack.

Terror follows close behind me
Sweat dripping down my neck.

Clenching onto destiny,
the weapon of my choice.

Striking rays of darkness,
wicked purrs of horror.

Lashing out with fury,
plotting my next move

As I refuse to give up
on a kitten fast asleep.

CHAPTER VIII

Risky Juggling

About The Poem

Risky Juggling is about having a surgery performed on my brain. When I first heard doctors discuss the idea of a biopsy possibly followed by the removal of something from my injured brain, I was both thrilled and terrified. What worried me the most was that – at the time – no one else had a surgery like mine before. Because my injury was near the brainstem (a delicate area that controls heart rate and breathing, which is almost everything you need to survive), it would be very unsafe to have an operation.

Poem

Risky Juggling

Round, round, round it goes
A chainsaw like a thunderstorm.
Engine roaring.
Blades thrashing.
Ready to destroy

Flames, flames everywhere,
a fire burns inside of me
Torches lit up,
matches burning,
searching for what is true.

Fear, fear, fearful thoughts
a possibility tossed into the air
Twirling around like a carousel.
Voices shaking. Hearts throbbing.
Never let it drop.

Sharp, sharp, sharpened knives,
piercing all internal thoughts.
Courage collapsing,
frowns emerging,
wondering what lies ahead.

CHAPTER IX

Balloons

About The Poem

After an operation on my brain hemorrhage (which was mistaken for a brain tumor), I woke up without any knowledge of where I was and why I was there. Consequently, I kicked and screamed; I was so rowdy, nurses tied my legs to my bed. Immediately after, my mom delicately explained to me where I was and what's going on. As a result, I calmed down and eventually fell back to sleep. When I woke up all the confusion and rowdiness somehow found its way back to me. *Balloons* is about waking up after surgery heavily medicated.

Poem

Balloons

Red balloons
Blue balloons
in the air I see balloons.
They look so neat from the ground,
I want them all for myself.

Yellow balloons
Green balloons.
I think I'd like some more balloons
The more I get the higher I feel.
I am so overwhelmed.

Pink balloons,
Orange balloons.
Nothing is better than these balloons.
I get an itch I cannot scratch
and so I squirm then start to laugh.

Black balloons,
White balloons
but who cares they're just balloons
When they deflate, I deflate
while insanity lies next to me.

CHAPTER X

Walking on A Tightrope

About The Poem

Due to my brain injury, my body became very weak, and I lost the ability to do many things. As a result, I had to have therapy almost every day. *Walking on A Tightrope* is about relearning to walk. At first, I thought learning to walk again would be a breeze. Unfortunately, I soon determined that I couldn't be more wrong; I had so much trouble balancing on my own two feet and would often plummet to the ground. Though relearning to walk was difficult, the real challenge was accepting that I did in fact once have a brain injury, and the disabilities that would stay with me forever.

Poem

Walking on A Tightrope

Thinking tall
Standing straight
Here I am,
I cannot wait.
Inch by inch
Step by step
Nothing to fear,
no need to stress.
The further I go,
the tougher things get
A constant struggle finding myself.
My knees ache,
My body shakes
Everyday my worries grow.
Walking in circles on a thin line.

CHAPTER XI

Wearing Clown Shoes

About The Poem

Wearing Clown Shoes is about the denial I experienced after much recovery from my brain injury. In the Fall of 2004, I began going to high school full time. Though I regained the ability to walk and was looking like my old self again, deep down inside I knew I wasn't. My classmates could do many things I couldn't, and it really upset me. Consequently, I often hid in the library, created the illusion as though nothing was troubling me, and ignored some of my friends. I pretended to be somebody I wasn't.

Poem

Wearing Clown Shoes

When chasing raindrops.
When chasing my shadow.
When chasing away the blues,
I will be parading in clown shoes
the sun's shining brighter.
Clown shoes, holding my chin up.
I think about hope.
I think about love.
Confusion consistently staring at me.
Clown shoes, tumbling and stumbling
Clown shoes, drowning in laughter
Singing all day.
Singing with passion.
Shrieking at the top of my lungs.
Clown shoes, dreams are suddenly better.
Clown shoes, nothing is softer.
Clown shoes, not quite my size.
No need to worry. No need to panic.
No need to be in a frenzy.
I'll often be dancing in clown shoes
the grass is looking greener.
Clown shoes, things couldn't be clearer.
Clown shoes, temporarily pleasing.
Clown shoes, nothing too appealing.

CHAPTER XII

Circus Express

About The Poem

Circus Express is about riding in an ambulance while feeling shocked and confused. In February 2008, I woke up feeling the same as I do every morning. When I came downstairs for breakfast my mom mentioned my face appeared to be droopy. I shrugged my shoulders, sat down, and started eating cereal. While doing so, I soon discovered that after every scoop I put in my mouth, the cereal would fall back into the bowl. At that moment, I was in such disbelief I repeatedly kept questioning myself whether this was a joke. About twenty minutes later, I arrived at a hospital and was diagnosed with the recurrence of my previous brain injury.

Poem

Circus Express

Zipping through town
with style and class
in a car so unique it drives in zig zags.
Clowns singing out loud
as the car turns around.
Honking the horn,
get out of the way.
Biting my tongue.
Laughter and fun.
Bouncing down the street,
speed bumps ahead.
A vehicle so pleasing,
a ride I won't forget.
A cotton steering wheel,
inflatable seats,
colorful belts,
everything's so fancy.
Driving offroad,
skeptical thoughts
There's no slowing down
in a car filled with clowns.

CHAPTER XIII

A Little Bit of Magic

About The Poem

A Little Bit of Magic is about having a dye injected into my veins. This procedure was done a few weeks prior to my surgery; the purpose of this was to determine the exact location of my brain hemorrhage. About half an hour before the injection, I was given medication to help me feel more comfortable and relaxed. This medication was so effective that I failed to realize when the procedure began and when it ended.

Poem

A Little Bit of Magic

Enchanted book,
enchanted cat
A rabbit pulled out of a hat.
Can you believe it?
Magic rug,
magic spell
Everything was going well.
So mysterious.
Purple cape,
purple mist
A show you can't resist.
Abracadabra.
Crystal ball,
crystal ring
You haven't seen a thing
too alarming.
Trick cards,
trick dreams
Nothing's what it seems.
It's an illusion.
Shrunken mice,
shrunken head
Conjuring up the dead.
Something special.

CHAPTER XIV

The Giant Elephant in The Room

About The Poem

After surgery on my brain, I had an unexpected stroke that left me paralyzed for about three months. As a result, I had to rely on several medical devices: a feeding tube, a breathing tube, an IV, and a few other things. Being paralyzed was extremely challenging; not only was I constantly bored, but I was often frustrated, confused, and uncomfortable. *The Giant Elephant in The Room* is about my stroke.

Poem

The Giant Elephant in The Room

Everywhere I look,
I see this giant elephant.
Standing in my way
Obstructing my vision.

Hogging the floor,
no room for the both of us.
Never have I thought
This could be such a pain.

Wherever I go
it's always close behind
Laughing in my face.
Please get away from me.

Falling out of place,
something to think about.
Though I see so clearly,
no one believes me.

Struggling to breathe,
gasping for courtesy.

Feeling insignificant
and I know who's to blame
Something so enormous,
nothing too elegant.

CHAPTER XV

A Timeless Trapeze Act

About The Poem

While lying in bed, the nurses frequently wheeled me to different parts of the hospital – no matter if I was asleep or not. I would often wake up confused in a different setting, and because I was on a lot of medication, I would make outrageous allegations as to how I got there. Eventually, as I gained strength, I was transferred to a Rehabilitation Centre, where I stayed for about five months. *A Timeless Trapeze Act* is about the various rooms I've been in while paralyzed.

Poem

A Timeless Trapeze Act

Freely soaring across the room,
far above my wildest dreams
Tightly clenching onto the stars,
knowing my heart will never sleep.
Letting go is not easy
even when someone's there to catch me.
Hands pointing towards the ground.
Life is turning upside down.
As I hold my chin up high
the crowd sings me a sweet lullaby
A dance performed in the sky.
Swinging with passion.
Feeling the love,
encouraging thoughts await.
Knowing I must always move forward.
When I peer down,
I wear a crown
made purely out of fear.
A thought will always rest in my head:
don't let the nightmares get the best of me.

CHAPTER XVI

Sword Swallowing

About The Poem

Sword Swallowing is about relearning to eat. Since I was unable to chew or swallow for a few months, I had to rely on a feeding tube which was attached to the inside of my stomach. Eventually, as I got stronger, I was eager to learn how to eat again and have this tube removed. At the beginning, I ate soft foods such as yogurt, oatmeal, etc. Eventually, as I began eating full meals, my dream of getting my tube removed finally came true. One day, two nurses entered my room, and a few minutes later, I glanced down only to see my feeding tube was gone.

Poem

Sword Swallowing

In the center of the stage
lies a sword shimmering with silver.
Immediately my attention is grabbed
as I hear my name drifting away in whispers.
While temptation begs me to have a taste,
I stop and think for a bit,
a strange request has been made
though strange has always been my friend.
With uncertainty all around me,
I feel pressured by my own thoughts.
With my mouth slightly hung open
I know time will not wait.
Still, I stall for a minute
bitter thoughts soon unfold.
Seconds turn to minutes
and hours never end.
Maybe tomorrow will be better.
I swallow down my pride.

CHAPTER XVII

Human Cannonball

About The Poem

Human Cannonball is about my first visit home after many months of being away from it. At the Rehabilitation Centre I stayed at everyone was allowed to go home on weekends. When I first found out about this, I was so excited and couldn't wait to go back to my house and sleep in my own bed. The first time I visited my house I rode in a bus with my parents because we weren't certain whether I could get into a regular car seat. When we arrived at my house, I soon discovered many things I couldn't do that I could before. My first visit home was not as sweet as I imagined.

Poem

Human Cannonball

Sparks of light
I feel the heat,
Now's the chance,
my time to shine.

What happens next
will be a blast
leading me closer
to the clouds.

Gaining speed
without a doubt.
Never have I felt so free.

A moment of shock.
A moment of joy.
My heart racing like a stallion.

When to stop?
I'll never know.
Only gravity makes that choice.

CHAPTER XVIII

Final Words

It has been many years since I had my brain injury. I wish I could say I'm now fully recovered and a stronger person because of it, but unfortunately, I can't. What I can say, however, is I'm a survivor of a life-threatening brain injury and though my life has been altered in many ways I have learned to cope with things. Every day, I am feeling more content with myself and though I still face many challenges, I am finally beginning to see a faint light at the end of the tunnel and that's what matters most.

The End

ABOUT THE AUTHOR

Jessica Wegrzynowski was born in Germany, has a Polish background, and currently lives in Canada. Since childhood, writing has always been a passion of hers. She enjoys writing short stories, poems, and songs. Jessica is currently an active member of The Tri-Cities Brain Injury Support Group and, in the past, has written several short blurbs with Michael Coss that were published in a magazine called Brainstreams. In December 2020, her first book, My Spring Fling: Young Love and Living Life to the Fullest, was published with the help of The Expert Author Press.